AMAALI LOKUGE

Amaali Lokuge is a practising emergency physician. She has been writing stories of patient encounters from the early days of her career. Her first story - "Phoenix" - about a patient's death after a difficult resuscitation, won second place in the 2006 Lorian Hemingway Short Story Competition. Since then, she has published short stories in several anthologies. During the pandemic in 2020, Amaali wrote for *The New York Times* about the Australian frontline experience and is currently a freelance writer for *The New York Times*. Through poignant, lyrical prose, Amaali illuminates the conflicting elements of tragedy, humour and absurdity within emergency medicine.

ALSO BY AMAALI LOKUGE

Fiction

A Doctor's Reflexes
in *Emergency: Real Stories from Australia's Emergency Department Doctors* (Penguin)

A Day in ED
in *Your ED* (Australasian College for Emergency Medicine)

How Many Cases Today, Dad?
in *When Minutes Matter* (Hardie Grant Books)

Non-Fiction

Racing Against the Virus from Inside Australia's Healthcare System
The New York Times

A Doctor Asks: Is Coronavirus Scaring Us Away from Our Humanity?
The New York Times

As a Doctor I was Skeptical About the COVID Vaccine. Then I Reviewed the Science
The New York Times

COVID's relentless Strain on a Melbourne Hospital
The New York Times

Where is Wellness Found?
in *Your ED* (Australasian College For Emergency Medicine)

AMAALI LOKUGE

TRAUMA

CRITICAL MOMENTS IN EMERGENCY

FENIX
PUBLISHING

FENIX
PUBLISHING
Melbourne, Australia

First published in Australia by Fenix Publishing in 2026
Cover illustration by Amaali Lokuge
Edited by Christopher Ringrose

A catalogue record for this book is available from the National Library of Australia

ISBN: 978-1-7647053-2-5

TRAUMA

CRITICAL MOMENTS IN EMERGENCY

1

She's asleep, but I have to wake her.

It is the morning shift, and she has already waited six hours to see a doctor. She rouses herself like a toddler, all puffy cheeks and listless eyes. Her skin is luminous in its softness. When she sits up and wipes the sleep from her eyes with the backs of her hands, she could be a portrait hanging in the National Gallery. But the light catches the bruises on her neck and the right side of her chest is distorted with the jutting bones of a fractured clavicle.

She has a sling for the fracture; analgesia has been prescribed already. I order a CT to make sure his strangling attempt hasn't disrupted the blood vessels in her neck.

But the important conversation is hanging in the air.

She doesn't make eye contact, impatient for me to leave. She has already been referred to social work. I ask her if she would like the contact details for women's shelters, whether she has anyone she can stay with. She shakes her head.

"No," she says. "I'll go back home. He's not like that when he's not drunk."

"But you could die," I tell her. "You're seven times more likely to die than other domestic violence victims who haven't been strangled."

She meets my gaze, holds it, seeing if I understand. 'I love him,' I hear her say behind that look. And in my eyes, she reads that I know exactly what she is trying to say. She's a piece of nickel by the side of the road, and he's an electromagnetic field the size of the MCG.

She will keep going back until she dies.

2

He had tripped while playing footy in the backyard with his grandson.

Just below the knee cap, his skin is tented, the fractured bone threatening to push through. His son paces in the corner of the room.

"My dad always says, 'If you do something, you have to do it well!' And I guess he's proven himself right," he says, as though clinging to the adage to hold himself together. The patient lets out a muted guffaw.

"I did pretty good huh, doc?"

I go to the computer just outside the cubicle to write up more pain relief and the nurse looks at me with wide eyes.

"Oh my god, that leg!" I exclaim, my eyes equally wide. There are more guffaws from inside the cubicle.

We move him to the resuscitation area to sedate him and reduce the fracture. As my colleague prepares the plaster backslab, and the nurse draws up the drugs, I check the airway equipment.

"He has a high-risk airway," I tell the nurse. "If we need to oxygenate, I will get you to squeeze the bag while I hold the mask." The nurse nods understanding immediately.

In the silence that ensues while we all get ready, the patient pipes up, "Hey doc, why did you say I have a high-risk airway?"

"Well, you have all that neck," I reply vaguely.

The clinical staff exchange looks. There is a suspended pause. Then the patient exclaims as though suddenly comprehending, "Are you calling me a fat bastard?!"

The room erupts with laughter, the patient joining in. My colleague almost doubles over, she's laughing so hard.

3

I call out his name in the triage room, twice. There is no answer. The clerk raps on the window to get my attention.

"He just went out for a smoke," she says, indicating towards the street.

The sliding doors open wide as I pass through, and a gust of wind brings in the smell of jasmine. Patients closest to the entrance turn their heads and breathe in the scent, temporarily alleviated from their problems.

I find him leaning against the wall, his right foot supporting his weight against the bricks, exhaling smoke rings into the sky. Passersby form wide circles around him. Maybe to avoid the smoke or to avoid him. He does seem slightly dangerous with his stubble, his nonchalant stance, and his ripped jeans.

He looks like he might carry a knife.

He stubs out the cigarette when I call his name and tosses

it into the curb. In one fluid movement, he lifts the canvas bag at his feet, slings it over his shoulder, and turns to follow me inside.

He has cut his forearm on a piece of metal. The wound is jagged, a V shape about 15cm long. It's fairly superficial, and none of his tendons are involved. I can close the wound myself without getting the plastic surgeons involved. I'm gleeful—suturing a laceration is my favourite procedure.

I prep and drape the arm and meticulously inject the anaesthetic. All the while, we talk about this and that. The medicine sorted, we focus on discussing life, falling into an easy rhythm of philosophy and banter. I laugh at something he says, drawing the thread through his skin and pulling the knot tighter. He flinches slightly when the needle catches a tiny part of skin that hasn't been anaesthetised. I apologise quickly, and he waves it away with his other hand.

"It reminds me of when I was in prison," he starts, then quickly checks himself and falls into an apprehensive silence.

"You were in prison? What did you do?" I'm shocked into asking and immediately wish I hadn't.

"Ha!" he says, but sighs and glances away. "You wouldn't want to know."

What would I not want to know? Rape? Murder? Is that what I wouldn't want to know?

I keep passing the needle through his skin. Delicate little stitches line up along the scar like fence posts closing off the bloody tissue beneath. I look up, and he has his head bowed as though observing the procedure, but he's watching me through his eyelashes instead. He's gauging my reaction, and I haven't even said anything yet.

I hesitate for a minute. But then I decide that it doesn't matter. In this moment in time, he is a good person who's letting me suture his arm and making my day lighter with his conversation. Thinking this, I smile with him.

He snorts, smirks, and then rolls his eyes up to the ceiling as though I am the most naive person he has ever met.

4

The nurse comes to me with the blood gas result, her eyebrows puckered.

"The pH is 6.9," she tells me with trepidation.

The patient is ninety-six years old. An acidaemia this bad will be hard to survive.

I go into the cubicle to see what treatments can be started to reverse the pathology. He is small and wizened, taking up just half the bed. His hands and feet are swollen with fluid from heart failure. His distended abdomen sits between his legs like a watermelon. He looks up at me with mute appeal, too weak to speak, just moaning when I palpate his abdomen and have a look inside with the ultrasound.

"She has to do that to see what's wrong," his wife reassures him, squeezing his hand between her palms. 'Please make him well, please let him come home,' I can read in the worry lines on her face.

"I think he's ruptured his bowel," I say to her and the nurse. I write up the antibiotics and fluids and order a CT. At least we will have a diagnosis to tell the family. I find a registrar who will be kind.

"Can you see this patient?" I ask, and I tell him the story. "I think he will be palliative in the end."

Later in the shift, I walk past the cubicle and can't help looking in. He is lying back, head bowed, sedated on morphine. She is still holding his hand. As I watch, she rests her forehead against his arm. I realise she is standing and only reaches the sides of the bed.

I imagine how they would have been just last week or the week before. Two tiny old people, walking slowly down the street holding hands.

I leave her to her grief without interfering.

5

I groan so loudly, the nurse asks me what's wrong.

"Aggression risk," I say, pointing at the screen. My last patient has only just been escorted out of the emergency department for swearing and yelling at me. I really don't want to be on tenterhooks trying to stay on the good side of another volatile patient. But I'm the only doctor in ambulatory care today, so I click her name and assign myself reluctantly.

She seems pleasant enough when I bring her in from the waiting room. Her toe is badly infected after a neglected injury to the nail five days ago. She flinches when I examine it, pulling away. She will need intravenous antibiotics and a washout in theatre, so I keep my examination cursory. As I stand up, I notice the beautiful tattoo on her leg.

"That's gorgeous," I tell her.

She eyes me, reading my face as if to see if I'm lying.

"I did it myself," she tells me with pride and melancholy mixed in her voice.

"Wow, you're an artist!" I exclaim. "So is this what you do? You're a tattoo artist?"

She sniffs and smirks with derision.

"Yeah, sure," she says. "If I wasn't too busy injecting ice!"

I grimace at her in sympathy.

"I know," I tell her. " Patients have told me it just takes one hit. The high is too powerful. I've told my kids never to go near it!"

She nods sagely and seems interested, so I tell her about my two boys to distract her while I try to find a vein. Her attention drifts, so I stop talking.

"I have four," she says. "Of course I don't see them anymore."

I look at her blankly. I don't know what I could say to make that better. I assume they have been taken away because of her drug use. Her pain bleeds into her eyes. But there is also acceptance.

The conversation pauses as I guide the needle into the skin.

Frustratingly, I miss the vein. She squirms and tries to pull away. I watch her apprehensively, wondering if she is about to reach her threshold of tolerance. But I manage to cajole her into letting me try again.

"Funny that you inject yourself, but you can't cope with an IV line," I tease her, now that I have better rapport.

"Yes," she says with a sigh. "My friend had to inject me the first time. I couldn't bring myself to do it. If only I had listened to my body and never done it back then."

Her body slumps and her voice is so full of regret I have to turn away. Like a coward, I busy myself with clearing the IV trolley.

Later in the shift, she is sitting on the orange chairs next to the admin area. Another patient has loudly voiced their displeasure at having to wait so long. I feel like shrugging and telling them to leave if they want. It's been that kind of day. Instead, I reassure them that someone will be with them soon.

I turn to walk into the computer room. She meets my eyes and gives me a little smile. 'You've got this,' she seems to say and it warms me to the core.

6

The cancer at the base of his tongue has been bleeding on and off. It needs to be cauterised before there is catastrophic haemorrhage. But there is no theatre space, so he will stay in the emergency department overnight. The bleeding has settled for now. Still, the registrar is worried, fearing the worst.

"I have everything ready if things go south," she tells me, fidgeting with the equipment, checking repeatedly that the patient is still stable.

"Go home," I admonish her. "There's not much else you can do."

The evening doctors leave one by one. The rest of us finishing later are having tea at the end of our shift, chatting and grumbling, waiting for the clock to tick over to 1am when we can also go home. The department is hushed. The nurses have dimmed the lights where patients are sleeping. The subdued aura of night shift is slowly replacing the frenetic pace of the evening.

The emergency buzzer peels and two doctors streak past towards resus 4. It's the patient with the tongue lesion. He's sitting forward, hosing bright red blood. A nurse holds a suction to his mouth and collects as much as she can. Within minutes, he has filled a whole sick bag.

Sweat drips from him and he looks at each of us with frightened eyes. I'm the closest on his left.

"It's bleeding," he mumbles through all the blood.

"Yes," I agree, distracted, checking the medications to sedate and paralyse him for intubation.

"No," he re-iterates. "It's bleeding."

The IV cannula has fallen out and venous blood oozes from the wound. He's losing a unit of blood every ten minutes from his mouth, and he's worried about the droplets running down his arm. But I bandage it up for him, and he seems relieved.

We are almost ready to put him to sleep and place him on the ventilator. But still, we hesitate. All that blood, the radiotherapy-thickened skin at the front of his neck, the distorted anatomy from previous surgery. After he's sedated, we may not be able to keep him alive. No one seems to want to make that call.

Sensing this, he turns to me definitively, grabs my forearm, looks directly into my face and pleads, "Put me to sleep now please."

"Ok," I tell him and call out to the team that I am going to start injecting the sedative. The plunger pushing the clear fluid into his vein, a silent prayer that it will all go smoothly.

7

She presents her finger to me as though the world is going to end. It's heavily bandaged and stuck down with multiple Elastoplasts. The triage note said, 'partial amputation of right index finger, dressings left intact.'

"Now," I tell her gently. "I am going to have to take the bandages down." She instinctively hugs her hand to her chest.

"You're going to have to let the doctor see it," her partner admonishes her, and she reluctantly places her hand on the trolley.

I have the anaesthetic ready for a ring block to deaden the nerves. But I need to assess the wound and nerve function before I can numb the whole finger.

Gingerly, I cut the plasters and expose the wound, watching her face for pain. She flinches with each unravelling, squirming in her seat, squealing when the crepe tugs at the skin.

Finally, the dressings are off. The finger lies limp on the trolley. All three of us lean in to inspect the laceration. There is total silence. The wound has closed over already. There is no amputation, just a cut that is already healing. Her partner laughs, head thrown back.

"But there was soooo much blood," the patient whimpers, looking up at her laughing partner for validation.

She wraps her arm around the patient's head and pulls her close. 'You're my histrionic weird one, and I love you,' the hug seems to say. The patient leans into the embrace, eyes closed, smiling sheepishly.

"I'm sorry to waste your time," a small, muffled voice emanates from the patient after a while.

"No, no," I say, taking off my gloves. "You've made my day!"

She doesn't realise the pleasure of having a laugh and an interaction devoid of the stress of making a diagnosis and the worry that you might miss something important.

I sit down at the computer to write her notes, and the nurse who has been listening in rolls her eyes at me. I just smile and enjoy the peacefulness of not having to think for five minutes.

8

He's cachectic and frail. The lines are deep on his sunburnt face; when he smiles, they form crevices around his eyes and mouth.

He is only sixty-four, and he is dying. The cancer in his oesophagus too widespread for resection, his body too weak for the radiation and chemotherapy.

He only has an infection today. He isn't in much pain.

"You know," I tell him while placing the cannula. "I worry about oesophageal cancer. Because I like to drink whisky and gin neat, and sometimes it burns on the way down."

His face collapses into those lines again as he grins at me.

"What?!" I blurt out, pausing the cannulation. "I'm being serious!"

"Doc," he placates me gently and asks how much I drink.

“A glass of whisky or gin most nights,” I tell him, guiltily. It’s my only vice; one I am loath to surrender.

Now he’s laughing at me.

“Doc!” he exclaims. “You’ll be fine! I used to drink a bottle and a half of whisky every night! And I’ve been smoking since I was twelve. I think you’ll be ok!”

He shakes his head, beaming at me. I seem to have made his day.

9

She is petite with silky white hair held in a bun at the base of her neck. The storybook grandmother, immaculate and neat. She had sudden-onset abdominal pain this afternoon, and now it is unrelenting and diffuse. Her stomach is tender all over, but not tense the way it would be with a perforated bowel.

"Where did it start?" I question her further. She gestures just beneath her breastbone where her pancreas lies. The tenderness seems most intense here too.

"Have you ever had gallstones?" I ask her—the most common cause of pancreatitis.

"What about medications?" She's not on any.

"What about alcohol?" I ask. But I assume the answer and barely pay attention to her response initially. She couldn't possibly have alcoholic pancreatitis. She doesn't fit my type.

"I like a wine now and then," she replies. But I notice the

way her eyes slide away from mine.

"Did you have some last night?" I persist.

She nods, admitting to drinking almost two-thirds of a bottle. She has had this pain before, just not this severe. She knows she shouldn't be drinking quite so much. It has never seemed a problem before.

"I think you have pancreatitis." I tell her, and write up morphine for the pain.

"Do you think it's from the wine?" she asks.

"It could be," I nod. "But we'll do an ultrasound in the morning and check for gallstones as well."

She grabs my hand and squeezes it. "Thank you," she says.

Later, writing her notes, I almost don't document her drinking. I want to let it pass, leave it as her little secret. How much harm can come of it at eighty years of age?

10

One of my colleagues asks me to sedate his patient in order to drain the abscess on his back. The patient is a prisoner; shackled to the bed. Two police officers stand at the entrance of the cubicle. An attempt at sedation with nitrous had been disastrous (as it sometimes can be), making him agitated and stressed, too tense to complete the procedure.

All rapport has clearly been lost.

I walk in and take over the doctor-patient relationship. Without that trust, procedural sedation never goes well. I check his mouth opening, ask about allergies, test the intravenous line, and hook up the monitoring. I'm a fresh face, a new person. For now, he decides to be compliant and amiable. I explain the drug that will sedate him, how it can sometimes create bad dreams. He's barely listening, so I start the sedation.

His eyes roll back when the drug kicks in. But suddenly he sits up in bed, tense and struggling, teeth clenched as though fighting someone away.

"It's okay, it's okay," I reiterate as I inject more sedative. "Just bad dreams."

He rests against the pillows with deeper sedation, but his muscles are still tense, his blood pressure high, his heart rate racing on the monitor.

"It's okay," I repeat soothingly, brushing his hair away from his forehead, the way I do with my children when they are distressed. Eventually, he drifts into a peaceful sleep. His heart rate and blood pressure settle.

My colleague extrudes pus from the abscess, holding the wound edges open, pushing the gauze deep into the wound. I see the patient's leg twitch and wonder if he is waking, in need of more sedation. I look at his face for signs of pain. But he is smiling slightly, eyes closed, feigning sleep. I realise I am still brushing his hair away. I seem to have forgotten to stop in all the drama. Embarrassed, I let my hand rest on the top of his head.

My colleague dresses the wound, and there is no more need for me. I go see another patient before this one wakes fully.

Later, at the end of the shift, writing up the sedation report in his notes, I remember the way he pretended to sleep as I brushed the hair back from his brow. I wonder when someone was kind to him—how long it has been.

His cavernous isolation seems to pass through the emergency department, a nefarious wind, taking me with it for a moment. The sadness hits me like a wave of nausea and I have to stop typing.

I lift my glasses and press the backs of my fingers to my eyes.

11

She has had multiple sclerosis for the last thirty-six years. She has been wheelchair-bound for the last eight. Her limbs are wasted and crippled. Her wife, her carer, is fitfully sleeping in the chair by the bed. The patient and I talk in whispers so as not to wake her.

They have been in the emergency department for hours. The shifts have changed and I have taken over her care.

She has an overwhelming infection, and her blood pressure is low and slipping. I was told that intensive care had placed a ceiling on her care. She is on maximal fluids and antibiotics—it's unlikely she will survive this.

I ask her if she is comfortable, whether she needs any pain relief.

"No," she says quietly and starts to cry. "How will she cope?" she asks me, nodding towards her wife. I have nothing to say to this. So I just hold her hand.

"You know," I say on a whim. "You don't have to give up. Your body could fight this if you wanted. You're on the right antibiotics now, and we've corrected your dehydration. I read an article that a large part of getting better is how willing we are to fight to live."

"I don't know if I want to live anymore with all this," She tells me. "But I can't leave her alone."

I give her hand a squeeze and go see the rest of the handovers.

Later in the shift, I place a blue tick against her name on the computer, alerting the nursing staff that she is ready for the ward. I glance at her observations. Her heart rate has slowed, and her blood pressure has lifted. I hurry to her cubicle before she is taken out of the department.

Parting the curtains, I poke my head in. Her wife is awake, and the patient is laughing with the her about something. She's sitting up, and there's a half-eaten dinner before her. Noticing me, she calls me over.

"See!" she says triumphantly. "You're right. I decided to live!"

12

I review his CT carefully before I remove the dressing. He's lucky; there's no vascular injury or extravasation of blood. Two bullet holes form neat circles on the underside of his arm, puncturing skin and soft tissue.

He peers at the wounds as I clean the area.

"Is that a 12 mil, do you reckon?" he asks me.

"I don't know man," I reply, shaking my head. "Bullet calibre is not my area of expertise." And at 19, it really shouldn't be yours, I think to myself.

"Yeah, I think it is. 12 mil. Heavy bullet. I'm lucky, yeah?"

This time, I think. This time.

13

I'm trying to reduce this patient's dislocated shoulder. There's a way to do it without sedation. But it needs patient cooperation and a lot of chatting about other things as distraction.

His dreadlocked hair and loose fitting, naturally dyed clothes remind me of the European tourists who would come to Sri Lanka for the surf. I ask him if he has ever been and we bond discussing my home country.

But still I'm struggling with the procedure, the humeral head stubbornly remains bulging anterior to the joint socket.

I go and get help from one of the other doctors. He also tries and fails. We decide to go ahead with sedation. The shoulder pops in easily and as the drugs wear off the patient sits up, groggily blinking his eyes, getting his bearings. I explain that everything went well.

He beams at me and says, "Isthuthi!" —thank you in Sinhala. It feels like he has been holding onto that word throughout the procedure, just to say it to me at the end. It takes me by surprise.

"Oh wow! My pleasure!" I exclaim.

My colleague gazes at the patient and then at me, trying to understand the sudden effusive delight flowing between us.

14

As soon as I feel the skin tighten beneath my fingertips, I'm certain he has appendicitis. I tell him straight away, so happy to have made an easy diagnosis despite his complicated story of recurrent bouts of pain associated with constipation and dehydration.

I'm referring him to the surgeons, and I start to second-guess myself. His blood tests are completely normal, with no signs of infection despite four days of pain. He has blood in his urine. I worry whether he has a kidney stone instead. The surgeons insist he needs a CT to confirm the diagnosis before surgery. I am starting to see their point.

I go back to re-examine him. I take the ultrasound with me to look at his kidneys and maybe, to see an infected appendix. His kidneys are fine, without any signs of an obstructing calculus. He has inflamed fat where the pain is maximal. I'm slightly reassured. But he can sense my doubt.

"No, doc," he says. "Trust yourself! You knew it was appendicitis as soon as you felt my tummy. You're going to be right. You're like a good mechanic. You know it when you see it."

I smile with him.

"We'll wait and see," I say.

"I trust you, doc. Stay fasting, right?"

I give him a thumbs up and leave the room. 'A good mechanic', I like that.

They take out his ruptured appendix later that night.

15

His wife has made him come into hospital. She had found him in the bathroom, an array of pills strewn on the floor, intoxicated, wanting to end it all.

He sits on the bed, legs drawn up, his forehead resting on his forearms. He has blown almost six times the legal limit on the breathalyser. I wonder how coherent he will be, but when I start the conversation, he engages with me as though he is completely sober.

He can't cope with the negative thoughts in his head anymore, can't stand the pain.

His wife calls, and we have a chat on speaker. Her photo on his phone is beautiful, a dark, charming-looking woman. He calls her baby, kid. She begs him to stay in hospital for her, to live for her. He tells her he doesn't think he can. I promise her that I will keep him in ED until he is safe to go home.

The patient and I chat for a while. The ED is quiet today,

and I have time. I tell him philosophies that have helped in my own periods of hopelessness. I try to make him commit to life, no matter how sad he is. He seems to be listening and taking it in, but counters most of my suggestions, saying he has tried them all before.

As a last resort, I ask him to imagine what it would be like if the afterlife is coming back as a ghost and having to watch his wife fall in love with someone new! In his intoxicated state, he turns to me, gives me a lopsided grin, but exhales a deep sigh through his nose. I suspect I'm trying so hard because I have just emerged from a similar, if less desperate, state.

During a pause in the conversation, he notices the way I fidget with my wedding rings, twisting them along my fingers the way the thugs in 1950s movies pass a silver coin along finger spaces.

"I do this all the time, sometimes I don't even realise," I tell him. "And my husband tells me off every time. He says he'll divorce me if I lose them!"

"I do the same thing!" he exclaims. "And my wife says the same thing."

He holds his hand out for them. I hesitate. What if he throws them and they can't be found? What if he swallows them out of spite? I have seen worse things happen. But I relent, and trusting him, place the rings on his upturned palm. I'm filled with trepidation, but I wait in silence to see what he will do. He runs his forefinger along the white gold circles and tries them on for size. They are much too small. He tries to pass them along, the way I just did, and fails. He gives them back. I run them down my ring finger and leave them there.

There is nothing left to say. We sit side by side on the bed, looking down at our feet, flat on the floor parallel to each other. He nudges my foot with his.

"I like you and everything you've said," he says softly. He bumps my shoulder with his, the way you would a friend. "But I can't stay, I can't do this anymore." And abruptly, he walks out of the cubicle. Shocked, I run after him.

"You have to come back!" I say in desperation. I promised his wife. He's not safe to leave in this state. He shakes his head as he lurches away.

"I'll call security if you don't!" I bark at him, switching to doctor-mode immediately. He turns slowly and looks straight at me. The sense of betrayal swells and amplifies in his eyes. I have lost his trust completely with those words.

But he comes back, and we get him to the locked ward. At least he is safe for now.

16

They're chatting lightly when I walk into the room—mother and daughter—an easy rapport drawn from years of shared confidences. They turn to me, laughing, and draw me into their circle. 'Just a check-up, probably a bad bout of gastro', I read on their faces.

But she has been constipated for ten days, unusual when she normally goes daily. Her daughter had found her this morning vomiting into the toilet.

"I made her come to the hospital. She had made an appointment with the GP," her daughter tells me, shaking her head. "For tomorrow morning!" she adds incredulously.

Her abdomen is distended. I see loops of dilated bowel on ultrasound—a clear bowel obstruction. But she has no reason for this, like previous surgeries or bowel perforations. It could be cancer at her age.

"It's a good thing your daughter made you come in today," I tell her gently.

"Can you be a bit more forceful when you say that!" her daughter admonishes me. "She won't listen to me."

I smile, and the patient smiles with me. I think she knows without my having to tell her.

Later that day, I check her CT results. She has a tumour in her colon which has spread to the pancreas. She is already on the ward. Someone else will have to break the news. I hope her daughter is still with her.

17

I am in charge today. It is up to me to maintain the flow of the department, to order tests, write up analgesia and antibiotics, and to clear the emergency cubicles by referring patients to different areas.

There's a patient on the 'waiting to be seen' list. A superficial self inflicted laceration to the neck, intoxicated. I look in on him to see if he is suitable for our behavioural assessment unit. I'm surprised to see he's the same patient from the week before—the one who tried on my rings.

He doesn't recognise or even remember me. I introduce myself as I would to a new patient.

I refer him for a psychiatric assessment and book the bed to move him to the closed ward. But I know it will be the same as last time. He will sober up and deny any suicidality. There will be no reason for us to keep him.

I hope I'm not on shift when he makes his final attempt.

18

I pull my puffer tight around myself as I walk out of the car-park. Fallen leaves swirl in circles and fly past my face. The chaos seems to reflect my inner state this morning. I bend into the wind, face down, gripping the bag at my shoulder, making myself walk faster towards the emergency room, hoping its clinical familiarity will provide some sort of salve to the turmoil I'm feeling.

I only have ten minutes before the shift starts. I'm worried it will not go well. When I'm in this mood, every patient encounter can be fractious. I promise myself I will get a coffee beforehand, as if to mitigate the risk somehow.

My first patient is a trauma call. He's been stabbed to the head and chest. The scalp laceration is the most serious injury, but we dress it quickly, and the bleeding settles. The anaesthetist and trauma doctor drift away when it becomes obvious that he is stable.

I prepare him for CT and go see another patient.

When I return to suture his wound, he's been moved to a smaller cubicle.

He is lying in bed talking animatedly to someone on the phone about the stabbing. A young girl, maybe his daughter, sits on a chair at the foot of the bed, and an older woman stands by the wall fussing with his bag of clothes. I bring the equipment to suture the laceration and talk him through what I will do while I get everything ready.

He seems happy enough to go ahead, so I think nothing of moving the bed down and setting myself up behind the head end.

I unwrap the dressing, and the wound edges begin to ooze. I draw up the anaesthetic quickly and explain what I'm doing as I start injecting. Scalp injections hurt like hell. I push the fluid in as I am withdrawing the needle to decrease the pain just a little. He starts to squirm and then to curse

"I don't mind if you swear," I tell him. "Studies have shown that it hurts less when you swear. But can you keep your head still?"

My tone is probably sharper than it should be; I don't seem to have my normal reserves of patience today. The suppressed frustration in my voice triggers him, and he jerks his head away violently. The needle is still deep in the skin of his scalp. I stop injecting, and he momentarily settles.

"Do you want me to stop?" I ask him.

"No. Keep going," he says through gritted teeth.

As I'm injecting the last few mLs of anaesthetic, he starts moving away from me down the bed. His hands are balled into fists, and veins stand out ropey and bulging on his neck. I glance at the woman for reassurance, but she's looking at the floor. The girl is watching her dad with fear plastered on her face.

Several things flash through my mind in succession. This man is probably a violent criminal in the real world, his family is afraid of him, I have trapped myself behind his bed and have just caused him significant pain. He hasn't threatened me at all, but from his family's reaction, I realise that he could probably turn on a hair.

"I might come back later," I tell him and start to take off my gloves.

"No. I. Said. Keep. Going," he says, with pauses between the words.

Not knowing how he might react, I don't really want to walk through the narrow space between the bed and the wall to get out of the cubicle. His daughter is still staring at him. I quickly staple his wound and dress it, grateful that the anaesthetic has worked so well.

Outside the cubicle, I lean against the wall, hyperventilating on the inside. I chide myself for so many things: that I didn't placate him better, that I didn't have an exit plan, that I didn't press the emergency buzzer, that I hadn't read the room correctly.

Later on in the shift, he's sitting up and relaxed when I walk past his cubicle. He meets my eyes and calls me over. Reluctantly, I stand at the entrance.

"I'm sorry I reacted that way, doc," he tells me jovially. "I was going down the bed, and then there was no more bed!" he exclaims, and laughs.

His family eyes me apologetically. Please don't trigger him again, they seem to be pleading. I decide to laugh with him—maybe out of guilt for my part in the interaction before. The tension in the room dissipates. He looks around at the woman and his daughter, proud of himself for making the peace.

19

His arm has swollen to twice its normal size, and the abscess is pointing at the vein where he injected ice two weeks ago. He will need to go to theatre for a washout.

He looks away as I examine him.

"Why did you wait so long?" I ask, curious.

"I didn't want my sons to know I'm using again," he says sheepishly. "And you're all so judgemental when I come in here."

I know what he means. I've been one of the judgemental ones in the past. It seems to be the luxury of youth to expect only perfection. I pat his shoulder conciliatorily.

"My uncle used to be an alcoholic," I tell him. "My mum and I detoxed him so many times, we almost gave up."

He looks up at me, listening. "And now he's been sober for years."

He shrugs. 'It happens to some,' he seems to say.

"You're meant to relapse—that's what addiction means," I tell him, gathering from what I've learnt. "But one day, it will be the last time. Just keep trying to stop. You haven't failed because you used this time. But it will mean it'll be easier not to next time. Trust me."

He smiles and nods. Maybe next time.

20

I am the triage doctor today. When the department begins to overflow, it's my job to allocate patients from the ambulance corridor to cubicles in the department or to the wards.

Suddenly there are ten ambulances and the department is full. I work fast to clear the area; there are always more ambulances on the way.

He's leaning over on the stretcher holding a towel to his face, a helpless middle-aged man, trying to stem the bleeding from his nose. I walk past him several times sorting out the other patients. The ambulance officer is with him and redirecting him to compress the right spot, but his eyes follow me, as though wondering why I'm not helping him.

'The other patients are easier to manage; I need a cubicle to deal with your face,' I want to tell him, but I don't. It doesn't seem right.

Finally, only he and one other patient remain in the corridor. I still don't have space in the department for him. I need to staunch the bleeding now. The other patient is delirious and half asleep; we have some semblance of privacy.

I have gathered the equipment and the numbing spray. When I take the towel away from his face, rivulets of blood seep around the crusted clot in his nostril and weep from the corner of his eye. He coughs up massive globs into the sick bag. I spray his nose and throat.

"There is no bleeding site for me to cauterise," I explain. "The only treatment is a nasal tampon pushed deep into the nostril."

He shakes his head in dismay when he sees its length. The blood oozes onto his hands, keeping time.

Finally, he agrees.

"The nose should be numb now," I tell him, asking him to lean his head back. The tampon halfway in, he jerks his face away and tries to turn aside. I know patients hate this; they sometimes refuse a second go. He's bleeding too profusely for an in-depth conversation. I place my hand on the top of his head and drive the rest of the tampon in. His startled eyes widen and stare at me in horror.

The bleeding stops immediately. But the patient's arms slump to his side, defeated.

"I'm sorry. I'm so sorry," I tell him repeatedly.

The ambulance officer with the other patient looks at me with judgement in his eyes.

It's another hour before I find the patient a cubicle.

21

She's beautiful with shoulder-length blue-green hair and a wistful smile—a prominent Adam's apple, the only sign of hormone therapy taken post-puberty.

Her collar bones encircle deep hollows at the base of her neck, and each time she breathes, the spaces between her ribs suck in beneath her tight white tank top. Her heart rate is 35, and her temperature low. Fine hairs stand up on her forearms even though it's a warm summer day.

"They thought I should probably come in," she says, leaning forward, her rigid posture unrelenting. "I probably haven't eaten in a week. Things seem to be getting out of control."

She sighs at the end of the history with an ironic arch of one eyebrow but remains tense and conflicted. I nod briefly and tell her I'll organise her admission to the eating disorders team.

"I have a lovely young lady with me at triage…" I say when the doctor answers the phone. From the corner of my eye, I see her smile to herself and relax back into the chair. Seeing me notice, her smile widens to include me.

22

I've seen five patients with chest pain today. Most of them are young. All of them have nothing wrong. I wonder if they don't have parents and grandparents to tell them about growing pains and muscle pains and just pains that will settle with time. But it seems the internet is more compelling, and every Google search of chest pain leads directly to death.

This boy is young too, just twenty-two. His mother has brought him into emergency today. His chest pain was six days ago. He is perfectly well now. No pain, no shortness of breath, no cough or fever. I feel ready to scream.

As he tells me his story, his mum stands next to his chair, feet wide apart, hands on hips, jaw jutting forward, challenging me to take him seriously.

"She went ballistic when I mentioned it to her this morning," he smirks, tilting his head at his mother.

"And why would she do that?" I ask, looking her way to

include her in the conversation. She purses her lips, itching to interrupt but making an effort to allow him to be the adult that he is.

He hangs his head.

“Well, the doctors always told me if I have chest pain, I have to go to the hospital.”

When I raise my eyebrows, he continues sheepishly,

“I have Marfan’s syndrome. My aorta is 4cm. The cardiologists are monitoring it.”

I kick myself for not having checked his file for past history before walking into the room.

I feel the familiar fear deep in my chest: this is a patient who could die. His aorta is dilated: I’m worried, and his mum is terrified, that it may have dissected six days ago. Nervously, I glance at his monitor. His vital signs are stable, and he looks well. I almost run to the ultrasound machine and drag it in.

He stares curiously at his heart displayed on the screen. The aorta is 5cm today. There is a thin layer of clot around the heart. The aortic valve leaks, and a dissection flap undulates ominously with each pulse of blood. I call the charge nurse to move him to resus and notify cardiothoracics and radiology.

"But I Googled chest pain from aortic dissection," the patient says softly. "It said the pain is tearing and goes through to the back. I had none of these, so I thought it was probably nothing."

His mother and I exchange glances and decide not to upset him with our judgement.

23

She has an extensive infection in her uterus and fallopian tubes—a complication of her work. It has probably been brewing for days. Her flushed cheeks blossom against her translucent skin, and she watches me through long, curling eyelashes as I organise her transfer to the Women's Hospital.

She smiles her thanks when I turn to leave the cubicle.

I hesitate, knowing I probably shouldn't. Then I ask her anyway if she's ever thought of doing something else.

"There are emergency ward clerk jobs going right now," I tell her. "I could get you an interview."

"Honey," she drawls with a smirk building on plump, lipsticked lips. "I make three thousand dollars on a good night. There's no way I'm doing anything else!"

24

He had been threatening commuters with a knife at the local train station. The police have brought him in. He was calm until the nurse told him he couldn't go out for a cigarette.

Now he's pacing by the side of the trolley, muscles tense, sweat beading on his forehead and chest. The monitoring leads have been ripped off. The intravenous line is on the floor. A bright rivulet of blood is lacing down his forearm. His eyes are bloodshot and protruding. The veins bulge in his neck. I hope they have already searched him for weapons.

Four nurses are standing two feet away, blocking the entrance of the cubicle. The police stand just outside. He is too intoxicated and erratic to be released.

He yells to be allowed to go outside for a smoke, for fresh air, for anything that takes him away from here. I stand there, unnoticed, taking it all in.

When security arrives, I tell him he cannot leave, matching his volume, but not his anger.

He turns to me and incredulous delight flashes across his face. I must seem easy to manipulate. But I stand my ground. I tell him I will have to sedate him to decrease the risk to staff and himself. He panics and backs against the wall of the cubicle. Suddenly broken, he waves his hands at us in opposition.

"Don't sedate me!" he yells. "Please don't sedate me!"

"But I have to," I tell him. "You're acting too violent for us to look after you."

"I'll be quiet, I'll be quiet," he mumbles and gets himself onto the trolley. "Please don't ruin my high."

At the end of the shift, the drugs have worn off and the valium has kicked in.

"Thanks for not putting me out completely," he says. "I paid a lot for those drugs."

25

She's presented today because her left hip aches day and night. She can hardly walk from the pain, but all the investigations from her GP have been normal. Living has become a struggle. She's eighty-eight years old.

"I even asked my doctor about VAD," she tells me. "He dismissed it out of hand."

"But why?" I ask incredulously. She just shrugs, trying to be resigned to her pain.

Not being my area of expertise, I sit down beside her and Google Voluntary Assisted Dying on my phone. The Victorian guidelines come up, and we read them through together. We both realise she would never be eligible.

"But isn't being eighty-eight a terminal disease?!" she exclaims in frustration, giving me a sidelong glance of defiance.

26

She was helped into bed by her son after falling against the dresser. This morning, she has sharp chest pains and is finding it difficult to breathe. When I see her, she is still quite intoxicated. She struggles to take deep breaths when I examine her chest, but doesn't complain. I wonder how much pain is being masked by the alcohol.

I suspect several broken ribs, and the X-ray confirms it. When I enter her cubicle to see if she would like me to block the pain with anaesthetic, she's talking to her son on the phone.

"I'm okay now, love," she says, tears sliding down from the corners of her eyes. Her voice trails off into a whisper as she struggles to contain her trembling lips.

I look through her notes, waiting for her to finish the conversation. She's fifty-four years old. There are no previous presentations, even though she lives in our catchment.

She agrees to the nerve block, and I get the equipment ready, chatting about this and that. I ask her if she has presented to other hospitals, and she says this is her first time in an emergency department. We fold back into silence as I inject the anaesthetic between her ribs.

The niggling feeling that something isn't quite right nudges at my mind while I clear up the equipment.

"Hey," I say, pausing until she looks at me. "Are you an alcoholic?"

Her eyes open wide and grow round with anguish. The tears seep from the corners again.

"I drink maybe four glasses of wine a night," she says, trying to keep her tone light, but her face betrays her. I watch her decide to own the problem.

"No," she shakes her head. "I'm lying. It may be a bottle. Last night I made cocktails. I may have had a few too many gins."

She turns her face to the wall and closes her eyes. I wait quietly, hoping she will engage again. And she does.

"That's why I'm crying," she whispers, cringing into the bed rails. "My son had to pick me up off the floor. I am so ashamed. "

"Don't be ashamed," I tell her. "It sounds like you've just slipped into drinking too much without even realising it. When did it start?"

"Not long ago," she answers thoughtfully, her mind casting back to the beginning. "I wasn't always like this. I think it started…"

"In COVID lockdown!" we both exclaim in unison.

I grin at her, and a matching smile builds on her face, breaking up the misery, the tension, and the regret. And for a moment, none of this seems so dire.

27

The police welfare check finds her in the bathroom, unconscious—a head laceration pooling blood beneath her forehead. Her clothes are torn, and she has fresh bruises along her inner thighs. She's emaciated and covered in older welts and cuts. The nurses gingerly cut the clothes away and dress her in a fresh hospital gown. Her head lolls, and we secure her neck with a hard collar. She is so small, so young, and so full of trauma. The mood in the room is deflated and miserable. Who would do such a thing?

The nurse and I go to the family room to talk to her mother. She is sitting on the couch talking on the phone. We walk in on the end of the conversation. There is a hint of carelessness in the air. She listens to our assessment, asks whether her daughter will wake up. I tell her I'm not sure; she hasn't had her head CT yet, I don't know if there has been any brain trauma. She nods. There is no emotion, no tears. Her indifference is chilling.

"This isn't the first time," she says. "The drugs, the boyfriend…" she shrugs and looks away.

28

She and her family have come down from Warburton for the Carlton game. Her husband and sons, decked out in team colours, fill the cubicle, looking on with worry for her.

She has tripped and fallen sideways, hitting her head on a doorframe. A 5cm laceration is oozing blood down her neck. The game is in half an hour, and she has no evidence of other injuries, so I quickly get the equipment to clean and staple the wound.

Her family leaves to find some food.

I've cleaned her scalp, felt under the skin for a skull fracture, and am just stapling the edges when I hear muffled sobs. Pausing the procedure I ask her what's wrong, but my concern only makes her cry harder. I put my arm around her shoulders and, leaning in, ask again,

"What's the matter? Does it hurt?"

"No" she whimpers. "I'm the only one who fell. I couldn't keep my balance. I am so fat and old." She shudders at the last comment, self-loathing filling her voice. I don't know what to say, so I pat her shoulder soothingly.

The procedure over, I hand over the discharge paperwork. Tears are streaming down her face and she makes no attempt to wipe them away. Her husband and sons avert their eyes.

'Mum is being hysterical,' they seem to say.

"Thank you for everything," her husband tells me, squeezing my elbow reassuringly.

Helpless, I watch her walk away—a middle-aged woman isolated in her distress at her changing body.

29

I am inserting an ultrasound-guided IV in someone else's patient. I don't know her history. But she seems fit and well. She reminds me of my mum—about 70 years old, I think to myself. I ask her why she has a carer with her; she doesn't seem disabled.

"I've had a carer since my husband died," she says.

I still don't understand. I lost my dad in 2020, and initially, my mum struggled to be independent, but now she's fine. The patient reads the confusion on my face and gets a mischievous look in her eyes.

"How old do you think I am?" she asks.

I lower my estimate by three years just to be flattering.

"Sixty-seven?" I ask hesitantly.

She chuckles, shaking in bed. I almost miss the cannulation.

"Eighty-three!" she exclaims, her face filling with glee and pride.

Just like my mother, I think. Still vain and delighted to be thought younger than she is.

30

The nurse sits at the computer, preparing to scribe for the trauma we're expecting. The cannulation is ready, the ultrasound machine is on, the pelvic binder is beneath the patient slide on the trolley. We stand around in anticipation, waiting. The nurse starts a story of a similar trauma, and it takes a hilarious turn. We all laugh; the anxiety dissipates.

The registrar moves towards the ultrasound machine. I look at my shoes.

The nurse tenses and shifts her posture. I follow her eyeline. Two tall young men loiter outside trauma 1. They're friends of my patient in 24.

"I've told you, you can't wander around the department. Go back to your friend in cubicle 24," she tells them. The boys bristle at her tone but pretend to be civil.

"Chill," one of them says. "We're just looking for the tea station."

She gives me a significant look and murmurs under her breath, "I have told them three times, that they can't be here!"

"The tea station is over there," I vaguely wave them away, hoping things don't escalate. They amble over to the counter, acting like they have just won a war.

"And don't come over here again. This isn't somewhere you can just stand around!" the nurse can't help saying. She's right, but I wonder if it was necessary.

"But you all can fucking sit around doing nothing?!" his retort comes fast and spiteful. We're waiting for a major trauma. It's our department, and the disrespect hurts to the core. The nurse deflates like she has been kicked in the stomach. It pains me to see her wilt.

I follow the boys to where they are standing brewing their tea. They seem at least two feet taller than me. But I am the most senior doctor on today, and it seems wrong to say nothing.

"You can't speak to my staff that way," I say. "You're going to have to leave."

Dumfounded, one of them turns to face me and argues loudly about his rights. His friend tries to pull him away.

"No," he states loudly, enjoying the drama. "I can be here if I want. Are you going to make me leave?" He swaggers towards me, towering over me to exaggerate his downward gaze.

I meet the charge nurse's eyes. "Call security," I mouth to her.

Hearing the commotion, one of the other doctors comes to my aid.

"Hey! You have to leave," she echoes what I have said and stands beside me for support. She is even smaller and slighter than me. He smirks, jerking his jaw at her, "You shut up, blondie," he sneers.

His friend takes a step back and looks on with trepidation. The entire department feels frozen. Patients, nurses, and doctors are all looking at us.

I'm angry now. I stand up on tiptoe to make myself taller. My voice involuntarily escalates to a higher pitch. My hands are shaking.

"You need to leave," I say as loudly and as forcefully as I can. But I know, I look and sound like a frail tiny woman. Briefly, I wish I were a man. Something about my tone, or my stance, or the anger flowing through me convinces his friend to try again and he succeeds in dragging him away.

Security arrives five minutes later. The department has gone back to what it was. There is no trace of the altercation or the stress.

31

She has been kicking and spitting, trying to get out of bed all night. The nurses in resus have had enough. She's not my patient, but the doctor looking after her is on his mid-morning coffee break. When I walk in, she pauses in her agitation to look up at me with big eyes, pupils dilated and cavernous from the drug overdose she took after breaking up with her boyfriend.

Suddenly sitting up, she pushes against the soft pillows buffering her from the metal bed rails and begins to climb out again. I go to her and put my arm around her shoulders, shielding her from a fall. She curls into me like a baby echidna, incoherently mumbling and slurring her words.

When I look up, the nurses are shaking their heads. They think I'm being too soft. They see a violent, self-destructive patient who has been causing chaos all night. I see a pampered, slightly spoilt little girl—what my daughter would have been if I had one.

32

The ring has been stuck on his index finger since he woke up this morning. The flesh is bulging on either side.

"I just got this yesterday!" he exclaims. "It wasn't so tight when I went to bed!" Frustrated, he paces next to the fast-track chairs, holding his hand away from himself. The student I sent to see him has had a half-hearted attempt at removing it.

"Cut it off! Please?" He says, thrusting his hand at me.

It's a beautiful ring, a dragon perched on his finger, its wings encircling the palmar side. I'd hate to break it. Anyway, it would take at least twenty minutes of grinding with the ring cutter.

I tell him we should have one more go at sliding it off. He shakes his head with distrust but relents in the end.

I inject the anaesthetic around the base of his finger, and when it's numb, I tease the ring this way and that, slowly easing it over the oedematous flesh. Finally, the dragon is free and in my hand.

I hold it out to him, enclosed in my fingers like a wild thing that may get away.

"Keep it," he says. "I'm sick to the sight of it!"

I drop it into my scrubs pocket. It plops in heavy and leaden—a kind of talisman.

33

Her hands and lips are blue, and she watches me with big, sunken eyes while I take handover from the ambulance officer. When I turn back to her, the nurses have already dialled up the oxygen, and her observations are back to normal.

She tells me her narrative efficiently, relieved that I have read her notes and understand all the complexities. As she is speaking, her vitality leaps from the bed. I can almost picture her out in the community when she is well, walking briskly down the street.

The chest X-ray is delayed, so I look at her lungs and heart with the ultrasound. The spaces between her ribs are pronounced with cachexia. She has large collections of fluid on both lungs, and her mitral valve is severely stenosed.

"That's much worse than it was last year," she says, watching the image on the screen, seeming to sense immediately the gravity of her condition. The blood passing through the valve has a velocity of 2.6m/s, reflecting the degree of narrowing. Her left ventricle is barely filling with each heartbeat.

I call her respiratory physician to organise an admission, and he highlights the futility of medical treatment for a case this severe and suggests end-of-life care instead. I persist and refer her to cardiology, advocating for surgical treatment of the valve, even if it only buys her a couple of months.

"She's not ready to die," I tell him. "Can't you do something?"

But her frailty, the palliative care plan from respiratory, the after-hours timeframe of her admission, all make the cardiology registrar dismiss my suggestions. Defeated, I downgrade her resuscitation status and go back into the cubicle to have that conversation.

The way she looks at me tells me she already understands.

"I know my condition is terminal," she tells me before I have a chance to stumble through an awkward explanation.

"I have made you 'not for resuscitation', if that's okay?" I ask, but actually I'm telling her there is not much more we can do for her.

"That's okay," she reassures me.

Her phone rings and she looks down at the screen before silencing it.

"They're all calling," she says. "But I'm not going to tell them to come in. I don't want to alarm them." She pauses before asking, "How long do you think I have?"

I dread that question. If she were to have her valve stretched with a balloon, she could have a few months. If we can drain the fluid on her lungs, she may go home with oxygen.

"Well, you're not dying right now," I tell her, glancing at her normal heart and respiratory rates. And, hoping the teams will change their minds when they see her, I add, "We may be able to get you back home."

"Yes," she agrees with me. "You don't know how tough I am. I'll survive this. I won't call them into the hospital." I don't contradict her, deciding to leave her with hope.

I look up her notes two days later while at home. I'm relieved that she has been discharged from hospital. But as I scroll down, I read her brief agitation, the hypoxia and cyanosis, the cardiac arrest attended by the MET call team. They didn't resuscitate her.

She passed away within minutes. She died alone. I wonder if I should have made her tell her friends to come in.

34

She's an eighteen year-old international student. Her flatmate sits on the chair beside the bed. Both of them are crouched into themselves as though loath to take up too much space. I've looked through her notes already: multiple presentations for this same thing—high sugars, insulin noncompliance, and dehydration—each time sent home with scripts and follow-up at our endocrine clinic. But the last note from the endocrinologists discharges her back to her GP after months of non-attendance.

She's a teenager. She was five years old when she was diagnosed with diabetes—I kind of understand the rebellion. Her sugars are five times the normal level today. Her kidneys are struggling. Luckily, she hasn't become acidaemic. I explain all this into their upturned sheepish faces and enquire if she has been taking some insulin. She nods mutely and allows her friend to take over.

"We ran out of the long-acting insulin she brought back from Dubai. We only have the short-acting left. We try to keep up with her sugars, but they keep going up and up."

"So how long haven't you been taking the long-acting?" I ask, confused. Usually, patients just stop all insulin, tired of the injections, the sick role. This doesn't make sense.

"About a month," she replies softly.

"She lost a lot of money to a scam; she can't afford to buy more. She has to wait for her parents to send supplies," her friend explains.

"So the missed outpatient appointments? You didn't attend because you couldn't afford it?!" They look at me blankly as though wondering why it has taken me so long to comprehend.

My heart tears slightly at its seams.

Outside the cubicle, I tell one of the other doctors about the tragedy of this patient. The cruelty of being unable to afford lifesaving insulin. He stares at me with steely eyes.

"But there are scores of Aboriginal children dying of the same thing every day. When have you been sad for them?"

His cold indifference is atypical, and I retort without thinking, "I would be sad for them if I saw them in my department!"

Immediately, I regret it. But it's too late. He raises his eyebrows and turns away from the conversation.

As I write the patient's history at the computer, the weight of what I have just said presses against me. If I could see them, I would care. Just like everyone else. The problem is hidden, so we do nothing.

Universal health care, we think.

35

She's ninety-two and has fallen from standing on the way to lunch with her friends. Her ruffled dress and elegant bag are laid out neatly on the chair. She looks frail and thin in the inadequate hospital gown, lying on her back in spinal precautions, a hard collar tight around her neck. A bruise is forming on her forehead and around her eyes. Blood thickens and tangles strands of her beautifully coiffed hair.

"I must look a real fright," she tells me.

I feel along her body for injuries— ribs, sternum, spine. She winces and catches her breath with each touch. When we roll her back, she senses my frustration that I can't pin down what may be broken.

She catches my hand as I turn to leave.

"I'm old!" she says. "Everything hurts when you get to my age."

36

She's had a seizure and is still post-ictal.

I talk to her partner to get some collateral history. She drank a bit too much with friends yesterday. The alcohol may have triggered this episode. She bends her arm in her drowsy state, and the intravenous cannula kinks, setting off the fluid line alarm. I try to troubleshoot and set off more alarms.

A resus nurse rushes in. Seeing me at the bedside, she brusquely asks what's wrong, silences the beeping, fixes the line, and walks out quickly. I grin sheepishly at her. Equipment has never been my strong suit.

"Who is she?" the patient's husband demands, noting the interaction.

"Oh, she's the resus team leader, one of our senior nurses."

"I don't like her!" he exclaims. "No personality! So rude!"

"Nah, she's fine," I placate him with a laugh. "She's just

efficient."

"Australians!" he keeps muttering. "I can't stand them. No humour, no fun!"

"But aren't you Australian?" I ask him.

"Of course not!" he says, deadly serious. "I'm from Launceston."

37

He's only twenty-eight.

'Increasing shortness of breath for the last six weeks', the triage note reads. No previous presentations. I check his chest X-ray before I go into the cubicle. His heart is twice the size it should be, and his lungs are fluffy with fluid. Heart failure. In a young person like this, it's usually viral, drugs, or alcohol.

He tells me he went to his local doctor when the breathing problems started six weeks ago. The doctor prescribed antibiotics and ordered a chest X-ray. But he never got around to getting the X-ray, never quite managed to follow up. He'd presented to other emergency departments twice but couldn't stand the long wait times.

He's breathing in quick, shallow breaths. The monitor reads thirty per minute. I tell him his diagnosis.

"It's the meth, isn't it?" he asks.

I nod and ask him how often he uses.

"Every day," he says, beguilingly honest. "That's why I never got back to the GP, why I couldn't get the X-ray."

Deep down, I know he will probably self-discharge at some point in this presentation—the call of another hit too strong to resist.

"But you have to stay with us this time," I tell him. "If you go home, you could die." He listens gravely.

I ultrasound his heart and it looms, dilated and ineffective, taking up the entire screen. He looks at it intently.

"So it's not working very well?"

"No," I tell him. "See this chamber, see how big it is, see how it's not contracting?" He glances away, unable to comprehend the severity of his heart failure.

I quickly place the ultrasound transducer just under my collarbone. My tiny heart takes up just a third of the screen and is beating valiantly.

"This is what your heart should look like," I tell him and then quickly fill the screen with his own heart. His eyes dilate with panic.

"I should just give up, huh?" he asks.

"No, no," I say. "Once we start you on the right meds, you'll be fine."

His goggles at me. We stare at each other for a moment in utter confusion. Slowly, it dawns on me that he's talking about giving up the meth, not life.

"Oh yeah," I say, giggling. "Definitely give up the meth!"

38

I have been called in at 3 am for a multi-casualty trauma call: kids joyriding in the middle of the night. Two have been ejected through the windscreen. One, a boy, is dead at the scene.

The streets are empty and eerily lit. Pools of light gather in circles on the asphalt, huddling together like homeless people. I've forgotten my ID tag and can't get into the car park. The sense of urgency quickens. I count the seconds at the red light of a deserted junction before turning back towards the hospital.

The only parking space is behind the police vans. Emergency vehicles only, the sign reads. I quickly scrawl a note and fling it onto the dashboard, hoping I won't find a ticket when I return.

The triage clerk releases the door for me and waves me through. I arrive just as the first ambulance rolls in. The overnight registrar is one of our best and has organised her staff into teams. Everything is ready to go. I'm almost superfluous, but my presence seems to reassure everyone.

I flit between each patient, overseeing, advising, helping with procedures. The sickest is rolled off to CT. The other one is stable and the doctors are dispersing. The third is screaming obscenities, refusing examination, pushing the nurses away, trying to get off the trolley.

She is only fifteen years old. She should be at the Children's Hospital, but sometimes we get the multi-trauma victims on the cusp of adulthood.

Her screaming increases in pitch and volume. I try to reason with her; first with entreaty and then increasingly with frustration. Briefly she pauses her theatrics to look straight into my face and yell, "Get out, you black cunt! DON'T TOUCH ME!"

I have only slept one hour since finishing the evening shift at 1am. I'm stressed that she doesn't have vascular access when her heart rate is 130 and her blood pressure is only 80. My resources are wearing thin.

"That's it!" I exclaim. "Call security, get some sedation."

The nurses trying to soothe her look back at me in surprise. 'She's a child! Her friend is dead. Give her a break!' They seem to chide me with their eyes. I realise I am making matters worse in the trauma room and drift into the background, allowing the more gentle registrar to take the lead.

The nurses spend a long time pacifying and coaxing her. The anaesthetic registrar on rotation from the Children's Hospital uses play therapy to get the intravenous cannulation. The nurses change her into a gown and she lets herself be examined.

I watch the interactions from the corner of the room, feeling small. In my haste and weariness, I had forgotten that she is only a frightened little girl, suddenly thrust into a cold and confusing adult world.

39

I sigh dejectedly writing up the notes of the patient I've just seen. A fifty-year-old mother of three with metastatic cancer; she's just two years older than I am. My colleague looks over at me quickly, concerned. Glancing at the screen, she sighs too.

"I know—it's heart-rending," she says soothingly.

"Fifties: the danger zone," I tell her. "My Ben's so worried about dementia."

"Is he doing anything about it?" she asks.

"No!" I laugh. "He just ruminates."

"I stress out about dementia all the time! I do my sudoku every day and my running. But listen to this!" she exclaims. "I saw this patient yesterday and his wife tells me, 'He's too confused to dress himself or get his own food, but he does his sudoku every day.'"

I stare at her for a beat before we both collapse into hysterical laughter.

40

He's been stabbed in the back and thigh. It's taken thirty minutes for the ambulance to get here, and now his blood pressure is unrecordable.

We got the notification twenty minutes ago, so we had time to prepare. I'm on for procedures. I have my scalpel and forceps ready to open his chest. I have checked the guide-wire and the dilator to get large-bore intravenous access. I have my sterile gown and gloves on. I stand with my palms together to keep myself from touching something inadvertently as they pull him across to the trolley.

The moment the ambulance stretcher is taken away, doctors and nurses swarm around him, doing their assigned tasks.

The trauma registrar opens the chest and tells the team that the left lung is up. I go through the cut already made by the ambulance officers on his right chest. It's too high, and the incision way too small. I extend it with my scalpel and dissect down to the ribs. Spongy lung nudges against my finger when I sweep inside his chest cavity. That job done,

I move to changing the small IV to a massive one.

"RiCC line is in," I tell the team leader.

He's dying, and the minutes are passing too quickly. It feels like we're running to pull him away from the precipice, but he keeps leaning too far forward. If only someone could reach him, grab his clothes, and pull him back.

My hands shake as I suture the line in place. My glasses keep sliding down my nose from the sweat. I nudge them up with my shoulder to keep them on my face. The blood is changed over to my line, and the nurse squeezes it in at high volume. But his blood pressure remains unrecordable.

I help the registrar with the ultrasound. The patient's heart is barely beating. Blood swirls and eddies in his right ventricle in a slow whirlpool. Everyone considers whether to continue the resuscitation. The team leader asks how much blood has gone in. My glasses keep sliding down. No longer sterile, I push them up my nose repeatedly.

We plan to roll him over to find the site of bleeding. The cardiac surgeon and trauma team discuss futility.

On the ultrasound screen, his heart attempts to beat every five seconds. The blood moves away from the ventricle walls and splashes back with each feeble contraction. Black streams of the fresh blood being pumped in circulate through the grey haze of his blood which is already clotting. I save as many pictures as I can—for teaching, for documentation. Frustratingly, my spectacles keep sliding down. The next time I push them up, the team leader calls out over the noise, "Amaali, will you stop touching your face! You're getting his blood all over your glasses!"

For an instant, the team pauses to look at me. Embarrassed, I make myself as small as I can. I don't touch my glasses again and pray they don't completely fall off my face.

Later, while the nurses prepare his body for the coroner, I collect the sharps from my trolley one by one. Reflexively, I lift my arm to nudge my glasses up and smile to myself, remembering: that tiny moment of care from my colleague, even in the middle of a colossal effort to save a young life from slipping away.

These are the stories
That linger
Replaying
Like song lines on repeat

www.ingramcontent.com/pod-product-compliance
Lightning Source LLC
LaVergne TN
LVHW050937210926
848482LV00013B/646
9781764705325